Contents

What is Renal Diet?

A renal diet is one that is low in sodium, phosphorous, and protein. A renal diet also emphasizes the importance of consuming high-quality protein and usually limiting fluids. Some patients may also need to limit potassium and calcium. Every person's body is different, and therefore, it is crucial that each patient works with a renal dietitian work to come up with a diet that is tailored to the patient's needs.

Below are some substances that are crucial to monitor to promote a renal diet:

Sodium

A main source of sodium is table salt. The average American eats five or more teaspoons of salt each day. This is about 20 times as much as the body needs. In fact, your body needs only 1/4 teaspoon of salt every day. Sodium is found naturally in foods, but a lot of it is added during processing and preparation. Many foods that do not taste salty may still be high in sodium. Large amounts of sodium can be hidden in canned, processed and convenience foods. And sodium can be found in many foods that are served at fast food restaurants.

Sodium controls fluid balance in our bodies and maintains blood volume and blood pressure. Eating too much sodium may raise blood pressure and cause fluid retention, which could lead to swelling of the legs and feet or other health issues.

When limiting sodium in your diet, a common target is to eat less than 2,000 milligrams of sodium per day.

Sodium is one of the body's three major electrolytes (potassium and chloride are the other two). Electrolytes control the fluids going in and out of the body's tissues and cells. Sodium contributes to:

• Regulating blood pressure and blood volume

• Regulating nerve function and muscle contraction

• Regulating the acid-base balance of blood

• Balancing how much fluid the body keeps or eliminates

Why should kidney patients monitor sodium intake?

Too much sodium can be harmful for people with kidney disease because their kidneys cannot adequately eliminate excess sodium and fluid from the body. As sodium and fluid build up in the tissues and bloodstream, they may cause:

- Increased thirst

- Edema: swelling in the legs, hands, and face

- High blood pressure

- Heart failure: excess fluid in the bloodstream can overwork your heart, making it enlarged and weak

- Shortness of breath: fluid can build up in the lungs, making it difficult to breathe

General Guidelines for Cutting Down on Salt

• Eliminate salty foods from your diet and reduce the amount of salt used in cooking. Sea salt is no better than regular salt.

• Choose low sodium foods. Many salt-free or reduced salt products are available. When reading food labels, low sodium is defined as 140 mg of sodium per serving.

• Salt substitutes are sometimes made from potassium, so read the label. If you are on a low potassium diet, then check with your doctor before using those salt substitutes.

- Be creative and season your foods with spices, herbs, lemon, garlic, ginger, vinegar and pepper. Remove the salt shaker from the table.

- Read ingredient labels to identify foods high in sodium. Items with 400 mg or more of sodium are high in sodium. High sodium food additives include salt, brine, or other items that say sodium, such as monosodium glutamate.

- Eat more home-cooked meals. Foods cooked from scratch are naturally lower in sodium than most instant and boxed mixes.

- Don't use softened water for cooking and drinking since it contains added salt.

- Avoid medications which contain sodium such as Alka Seltzer and Bromo Seltzer.

- For more information; food composition books are available which tell how much sodium is in food.

Meats, Poultry, Fish, Legumes, Eggs and Nuts

High-Sodium Foods

- Smoked, cured, salted or canned meat, fish or poultry including bacon, cold cuts, ham, frankfurters, sausage, sardines, caviar and anchovies

- Frozen breaded meats and dinners, such as burritos and pizza

- Canned entrees, such as ravioli, spam and chili

- Salted nuts

- Beans canned with salt added

Low-Sodium Alternatives

- Any fresh or frozen beef, lamb, pork, poultry and fish

- Eggs and egg substitutes

- Low-sodium peanut butter

- Dry peas and beans (not canned)

- Low-sodium canned fish

- Drained, water or oil packed canned fish or poultry

Dairy Products

High-Sodium Foods

- Buttermilk

- Regular and processed cheese, cheese spreads and sauces

- Cottage cheese

Low-Sodium Alternatives

- Milk, yogurt, ice cream and ice milk

- Low-sodium cheeses, cream cheese, ricotta cheese and mozzarella

Breads, Grains and Cereals

High-Sodium Foods

- Bread and rolls with salted tops

- Quick breads, self-rising flour, biscuit, pancake and waffle mixes

- Pizza, croutons and salted crackers

- Prepackaged, processed mixes for potatoes, rice, pasta and stuffing

Low-Sodium Alternatives

- Breads, bagels and rolls without salted tops

- Muffins and most ready-to-eat cereals

- All rice and pasta, but do not to add salt when cooking

- Low-sodium corn and flour tortillas and noodles

- Low-sodium crackers and breadsticks

- Unsalted popcorn, chips and pretzels

Vegetables and Fruits

High-Sodium Foods

- Regular canned vegetables and vegetable juices

- Olives, pickles, sauerkraut and other pickled vegetables

- Vegetables made with ham, bacon

- Packaged mixes, such as scalloped or au gratin potatoes, frozen hash browns and Tater Tots

- Commercially prepared pasta and tomato sauces and salsa

Low-Sodium Alternatives

- Fresh and frozen vegetables without sauces

- Low-sodium canned vegetables, sauces and juices

- Fresh potatoes, frozen French fries and instant mashed potatoes

- Low-salt tomato or V-8 juice.

- Most fresh, frozen and canned fruit

- Dried fruits

Soups

High-Sodium Foods

- Regular canned and dehydrated soup, broth and bouillon

- Cup of noodles and seasoned ramen mixes

Low-Sodium Alternatives

- Low-sodium canned and dehydrated soups, broth and bouillon

- Homemade soups without added salt

Fats, Desserts and Sweets

High-Sodium Foods

- Soy sauce, seasoning salt, other sauces and marinades

- Bottled salad dressings, regular salad dressing with bacon bits

- Salted butter or margarine

- Instant pudding and cake

- Large portions of ketchup, mustard

Low-Sodium Alternatives

- Vinegar, unsalted butter or margarine

- Vegetable oils and low sodium sauces and salad dressings

- Mayonnaise

- All desserts made without salt

Potassium

Every time you eat a banana or a baked potato with the skin on (not just the tasty buttered insides), you're getting potassium. This essential mineral keeps your muscles healthy and your heartbeat and blood pressure steady.

If you have a heart or kidney condition, though, your doctor may recommend a low-potassium diet. Your kidneys are responsible for keeping a healthy amount of potassium in your body. If they're not working right, you may get too much or too little.

If you have too much potassium in your blood, it can cause cardiac arrest -- when your heart suddenly stops beating.

If you have too little potassium in your blood, it can cause an irregular heartbeat. Your muscles may also feel weak.

What is Potassium and its role in the body?

Potassium is a mineral found in many of the foods we eat and is also found naturally in the body. Potassium plays a role in keeping the heartbeat regular and the muscles working correctly. Potassium is also necessary for maintaining fluid and electrolyte balance in the bloodstream. The kidneys help to keep the right amount of potassium in your body and they expel excess amounts into the urine.

Why should kidney patients monitor their potassium intake?

When the kidneys fail, they can no longer remove excess potassium, so potassium levels build up in the body. High potassium in the blood is called hyperkalemia which can cause:

- Muscle weakness

- An irregular heart beat

- Slow pulse

- Heart attacks

- Death

How can patients monitor their potassium intake?

When the kidneys no longer regulate potassium, a patient must monitor the amount of potassium that enters the body.

Tips to help keep the levels of potassium in your blood safe, make sure to:

• Talk with a renal dietitian about creating an eating plan.

• Limit foods that are high in potassium.

• Limit milk and dairy products to 8 oz per day.

• Choose fresh fruits and vegetables.

• Avoid salt substitutes & seasonings with potassium.

- Read labels on packaged foods & avoid potassium chloride.

- Pay close attention to serving size.

- Keep a food journal.

High-Potassium Foods

Most foods have potassium. To keep your levels low, avoid or eat less than a half-cup a day of these high-potassium foods:

High-potassium fruits:

- Apricots

- Bananas

- Cantaloupe

- Dried fruit

- Honeydew melon

- Kiwi

- Mango

- Nectarines

- Oranges and orange juice

- Papaya

- Pomegranate and pomegranate juice

- Prunes and prune juice

- Pumpkin

- Raisins

High-potassium vegetables:

- Acorn squash, butternut squash, Hubbard squash

- Avocado

- Artichoke

- Beets

- Baked beans, black beans, refried beans

- Broccoli (cooked)

- Brussels sprouts

- Kohlrabi

- Lentils

- Okra

- Onions (fried)

- Parsnips

- Potatoes (white and sweet)

- Rutabagas

- Spinach (cooked)

- Tomatoes, tomato sauce, and tomato paste

- Vegetable juice

Other high-potassium foods:

- Bran products

- Chocolate

- Coconut

- Creamed soups

- French fries

- Granola

- Ice cream

- Milk (buttermilk, chocolate, eggnog evaporated, malted, soy and milkshakes)

- Miso

- Molasses

- Nuts

- Peanut butter

- Potato chips

- Salt substitutes

- Seeds

- Tofu

- Yogurt

Low-Potassium Foods

The list of high-potassium foods may feel a bit overwhelming, but remember, for every high-potassium food to avoid, there's at least one low-potassium food to enjoy.

The recommended serving size for these low-potassium foods is 1/2 cup. You don't want to overdo it. Too much of a low-potassium food makes it a high-potassium food.

Low-potassium fruits:

• Apples (plus apple juice and applesauce)

• Blackberries

• Blueberries

• Cranberries

• Fruit cocktail

• Grapes and grape juice

• Grapefruit

• Mandarin oranges

• Peaches

* Pears

* Pineapple and pineapple juice

* Plums

* Raspberries

* Strawberries

* Tangerine

* Watermelon

Low-potassium vegetables:

* Alfalfa sprouts

* Asparagus (6 raw spears)

* Broccoli (raw or cooked from frozen)

* Cabbage

* Carrots (cooked)

- Cauliflower

- Celery (1 stalk)

- Corn (half an ear if it's on the cob)

- Cucumber

- Eggplant

- Green beans or wax beans

- Kale

- Lettuce

- White mushrooms (raw)

- Onion

- Parsley

- Peas (green)

- Peppers

- Radish

- Water chestnuts

- Watercress

- Yellow squash and zucchini

Other low-potassium foods:

- Bread (not whole grain)

- Cake (angel or yellow)

- Coffee (8 ounces)

- Cookies (no nuts or chocolate)

- Noodles

- Pasta

- Pies (no chocolate or high-potassium fruit)

- Rice

- Tea (16 ounces max)

Here's a trick: You can lower the potassium levels in certain vegetables by a cooking process called leaching. Try this on white and sweet potatoes, carrots, beets, winter squash, and rutabagas.

Fill a pot with warm water. Peel your vegetable and rinse it in warm water, then cut it into 1/8th-inch-thick slices. Rinse the slices and soak them in the pot for 2 hours. When you pull them out, rinse them again with warm water. Drain the water in the pot, fill it again, and cook your vegetable.

If you want to leach more than one vegetable at a time, soak them in 10 times the amount of water to the amount of vegetables. And when you cook them, use five times more water than vegetables.

Based on the amount of potassium that's right for you, ask your doctor or nutritionist how to balance high- and low-potassium foods in each meal.

Phosphorus

There are several nutrients that should be kept in check when you are dealing with kidney disease. In particular, phosphorus is a mineral that is important for many body functions. It is found in your bones and helps your body build cells and helps energy transfers throughout the cells. When kidneys are working normally, they remove extra phosphorus in the blood. But, when your kidneys aren't working well, your body is not able to get rid of the extra phosphorus. Having too much phosphorus can affect the balance of other minerals in your blood. A specific balance between the amount of calcium and the amount of phosphorus is vital. If the extra phosphorus cannot be released from your body, it will build up in your blood. This buildup causes calcium to be pulled from your bones in an effort to regain that needed balance. If too much calcium is pulled, your bones may become brittle and weak.

What is Phosphorus and its role in the body?

Phosphorus is a mineral that is critical in bone maintenance and development. Phosphorus also assists in the development of connective tissue and organs and aids in muscle movement. When food containing phosphorus is consumed and digested, the small intestines absorb the phosphorus so that it can be stored in the bones.

Why should kidney patients monitor Phosphorus intake?

Normal working kidneys can remove extra phosphorus in your blood. When kidney function is compromised, the kidneys no longer remove excess phosphorus. High phosphorus levels can pull calcium out of your bones, making them weak. This also leads to dangerous calcium deposits in the blood vessels, lungs, eyes, and heart.

How can patients monitor their Phosphorus intake?

Phosphorus can be found in many foods. Therefore, patients with compromised kidney function should work with a renal dietitian to help manage phosphorus levels.

Tips to help keep phosphorus at safe levels:

• Know what foods are lower in phosphorus.

• Pay close attention to serving size

• Eat smaller portions of foods that are high in protein at meals and for snacks.

• Eat fresh fruits and vegetables.

• Ask your physician about using phosphate binders at meal time.

- Avoid packaged foods that contain added phosphorus. Look for phosphorus, or for words with "PHOS" on ingredient labels.

- Keep a food journal

Lower-Phosphorus Alternatives to Choose:

- Fresh fruits and vegetables

- Rice milk, unenriched

- Breads

- Pasta

- Rice

- Fish

- Corn and rice cereals

- Soda without phosphate additives

- Home-brewed ice tea

High Phosphorus Foods to Avoid or Limit:

- Dairy foods

- Beans

- Lentils

- Nuts

- Bran cereals

- Oatmeal

- Colas and other drinks with phosphate additives

- Some bottled ice tea

Some foods may also contain phosphate additives that could add up to 1000 mg/day of phosphorus to your diet. Since you have likely been asked by your doctor to limit your phosphorous to 800-1000mg/day, these are additives you should be aware of. Some foods that contain these additives are:

- Processed meats

- Instant puddings and sauces

- Spreadable cheeses

- Beverage products

Protein

Protein is not a problem for healthy kidneys. Normally, protein is ingested and waste products are created, which in turn are filtered by the nephrons of the kidney. Then, with the help of additional renal proteins, the waste turns into urine. In contrast, damaged kidneys fail to remove protein waste and it accumulates in the blood.

The proper consumption of protein is tricky for Chronic Kidney Disease patients as the amount differs with each stage of disease. Protein is essential for tissue maintenance and other bodily roles, so it is important to eat the recommended amount for the specific stage of disease according to your nephrologist or renal dietician.

Low-protein foods

The following are low-protein foods:

• all fruits, except dried fruits

• all vegetables, except peas, beans, and corn

• many sources of healthful fats, such as olive oil and avocados

• herbs and spices

Many other types of food are low in protein, and a person should use moderation when incorporating them into the diet. Some of these foods include:

• sugar

• candies that do not contain gelatin

• tea and coffee, without dairy milk

- jams and jellies

- mayonnaise

- butter

- many sauces and dressings, including tomato sauces and salad dressings

Moderate-protein foods

On a low-protein diet, people should eat foods that contain moderate amounts of protein sparingly. Examples include:

- bread

- crackers

- breakfast cereals

- pasta

- oats

- corn

- rice

Fluids

Fluid control is important for patients in the later stages of Chronic Kidney Disease because normal fluid consumption may cause fluid build up in the body which could become dangerous. People on dialysis often have decreased urine output, so increased fluid in the body can put unnecessary pressure on the person's heart and lungs.

A patient's fluid allowance is calculated on an individual basis, depending on urine output and dialysis settings. It is vital to follow your nephrologist's/nutritionist's fluid intake guidelines.

To control fluid intake, patients should:

• Not drink more than what your doctor orders

• Count all foods that will melt at room temperature (Jell-O®, popsicles, etc.)

• Be cognizant of the amount of fluids used in cooking

RENAL DIET RECIPES

Trying new kidney-friendly recipes is a great way to explore new flavors and find new favorite dishes while looking after your health. In this part are nourishing renal diet recipes

Southwest Baked Egg Breakfast Cups

Preparation time

25 minutes

Ingredients

* 3 cups rice, cooked

* 4 ounces cheddar cheese, shredded

* 4 ounces green chilies, diced

* 2 ounces pimentos, drained and diced

* ½ cup skim milk

* 2 eggs, beaten

* ½ teaspoon ground cumin

* ½ teaspoon black pepper

- nonstick cooking spray

Instructions

1. In a large bowl, combine rice, 2 ounces of cheese, chilies, pimentos, milk, eggs, cumin and pepper.

2. Spray muffin cups with nonstick cooking spray.

3. Spoon mixture evenly into 12 muffin cups.

4. Sprinkle top of each cup with the remaining 2 ounces of shredded cheese.

5. Bake at 400° F for 15 minutes or until set.

Blueberry Muffins

Preparation time

45 minutes

Ingredients

- ½ cup unsalted butter

- 1 ¼ cups sugar

- 2 eggs

- 2 cups 1% milk

- 2 cups all-purpose flour

- 2 teaspoons baking powder

- ½ teaspoon salt

- 2 ½ cups fresh blueberries

- 2 teaspoons sugar (for topping)

Instructions

1. Using a mixer set on low speed, blend margarine and sugar until creamy and fluffy.

2. Add eggs one at a time and mix until blended.

3. Sift dry ingredients and add alternately with milk.

4. Mash ½ cup blueberries and stir in by hand. Then add remaining blueberries and stir in by hand.

5. Spray muffin cups and surface of pan with vegetable oil. Place muffins cups in tin.

6. Pile muffin mixture high in each muffin cup. Sprinkle sugar over muffin tops.

7. Bake at 375° F for 25–30 minutes. Cool in pan for at least 30 minutes before removing carefully.

Easy Turkey Breakfast Burritos

Preparation time

30 minutes

Ingredients

- 1 pound of ground turkey or use 1 pound leftover turkey meatloaf, cubed small

- 8 6-inch flour burrito shells

- ¼ cup canola oil

- 8 beaten eggs, scrambled

- ¼ cup diced onions

- ¼ cup fresh bell peppers (red, yellow or green), diced

- 2 tablespoons seeded jalapeño peppers

- 2 tablespoons fresh scallions, chopped

- 2 tablespoons fresh cilantro, chopped

- ½ teaspoon chili powder

- ½ teaspoon smoked paprika

- 1 cup shredded Monterey Jack and Cheddar cheese

Instructions

1. Sauté meatloaf, onions, peppers, scallions and cilantro in half the oil until translucent.

2. Stir in spices and then turn off heat.

3. Using another large sauté pan, set pan to medium-high heat and add in remaining oil and scrambled eggs.

4. Place equal amounts of vegetable and meatloaf mix, cheese and eggs in burrito shells, then fold and serve.

Spicy Tofu Scrambler

Preparation time

35 minutes

Ingredients

- 1 teaspoon olive oil

- ¼ cup red bell pepper, chopped

- ¼ cup green bell pepper, chopped

- 1 cup firm tofu (choose less than 10% calcium)

- 1 teaspoon onion powder

- ¼ teaspoon garlic powder

- 1 clove garlic, minced

- ⅛ teaspoon turmeric

Instructions

1. In a medium-sized, nonstick skillet, sauté garlic and both bell peppers in olive oil.

2. Rinse and drain tofu and crumble it into the skillet.

3. Add the remaining ingredients.

4. Stir and cook on low to medium heat until the tofu turns a slight golden brown, about 20 minutes.

5. Water will evaporate out of the mixture.

6. Serve tofu scrambler warm.

Cheesesteak Quiche

Preparation time

1 hour

Ingredients

- ½ pound shaved sirloin steak meat, coarsely chopped

- 1 cup onions, diced

- 2 tablespoons canola oil

- ½ cup pepper jack cheese, shredded

- 5 eggs, beaten

- 1 cup cream

- 1" x 9" deep par-cooked prepared piecrust*

- ½ teaspoon ground black pepper

Instructions

1. Chop the shaved sirloin into coarse pieces.

2. Sauté chopped steak and onions in a sauté pan with oil until meat is browned through.

3. Set aside to cool slightly for 10 minutes.

4. Fold in cheese and let sit.

5. In a large bowl, beat eggs and cream together with black pepper until thoroughly mixed.

6. Spread steak and cheese mix onto bottom of par-cooked piecrust, then pour egg mixture over the top and bake at 350° F for 30 minutes.

7. Cover cheesesteak quiche with foil and turn off oven. Let the quiche set for 10 minutes, then serve.

Chocolate Pancakes With Moon Pie Stuffing

Preparation time

30 minutes

Ingredients

Moon Pie Stuffing:

- 1 tablespoon unsweetened cocoa powder

- ¼ cup heavy cream

- ½ cup cream cheese, softened

- ½ cup marshmallow cream

Chocolate Pancakes:

- 1 cup flour

- 3 tablespoons sugar

- 3 tablespoons unsweetened cocoa powder

- ½ teaspoon baking soda

- 1 tablespoon lemon juice

- 1 egg

- 1 cup 2% milk

- 2 tablespoons canola oil

- 2 teaspoons vanilla extract

- 2/3 cup Body Fortress® vanilla whey protein powder

Instructions

Moon Pie Filling:

1. Beat cocoa and heavy cream together until stiff peaks are formed.

2. Whip in cream cheese, marshmallow cream and whey protein powder for about a minute or until well blended, but don't overbeat.

3. Cover and set aside in fridge.

Pancakes:

1. Mix all the dry ingredients together in a large bowl and set aside.

2. Mix all the wet ingredients in medium-size bowl.

3. Slowly fold in wet ingredients to the dry ingredients just until wet, but don't over mix.

4. Cook the pancakes on a lightly oiled griddle on medium heat or 375° F.

5. Use about 1/8 cup of batter to form 4-inch pancakes, flipping when they start to bubble

Fluffy Homemade Buttermilk Pancakes

Preparation time

20 minutes

Ingredients

- 2 cups all-purpose flour

- 1 teaspoon cream of tartar

- 1½ teaspoons baking soda

- 2 tablespoons sugar

- 2 cups low-fat buttermilk

- 2 large eggs

- ¼ cup canola oil and 1 tablespoon canola oil (for cooking)

Instructions

Warm up a skillet on medium heat.

1. Combine dry ingredients in a large bowl.

2. Add dry ingredients to buttermilk, oil and egg mixture.

3. Use a whisk or spoon to blend the dry ingredients until they are completely moist.

4. Use a tablespoon of canola oil to grease the skillet.

5. Using a ⅓-cup measuring cup, scoop the pancake mixture on the skillet. Each pancake should spread to about 4 inches across.

6. Leave about 2" between the pancakes for easy flipping.

7. Flip pancakes using a spatula—do this when the bubbles on the top of the pancakes have mostly disappeared. Allow the other side to brown until the center no longer appears wet.

8. Move to serving dish.

For a healthier twist, think of serving with fresh berries and a side of eggs.

Lemon Orzo Spring Salad

Preparation time

30 minutes

Ingredients

- ¾ cup or ¼ box orzo pasta

- ¼ cup fresh yellow peppers, diced

- ¼ cup fresh red peppers, diced

- ¼ cup fresh green peppers, diced

- ½ cup fresh red or Vidalia onion, diced

- 2 cups fresh zucchini, medium-cubed

- ¼ cup and 2 tablespoons olive oil

- 3 tablespoons fresh lemon juice

- 1 teaspoon lemon zest

- 3 tablespoons grated Parmesan cheese

- 2 tablespoons fresh rosemary, chopped

- ½ teaspoon black pepper

- ½ teaspoon dried oregano

- ½ teaspoon red pepper flakes

Instructions

1. Cook orzo pasta according to box directions, drain and let sit. (Do not rinse.)

2. Sauté peppers, onions and zucchini on medium-high heat with 2 tablespoons of oil in large pan until translucent.

3. Mix lemon juice, lemon zest, ¼ cup olive oil, cheese, rosemary, pepper, oregano and red pepper flakes in a large bowl.

4. Add sautéed vegetables and orzo pasta into the large bowl and fold gently until well mixed.

5. Chill or serve at room temperature

Chilled Veggie and Shrimp Noodle Salad

Preparation time

15 minutes

Ingredients

- 1 pound package of dry Spaghetti, noodles cooked and chilled (don't rinse)

- 4 cups cooked cocktail shrimp, peeled, deveined, tailless and cut in half; or 14-ounce pack of cooked salad shrimp

- 1 cup fresh scallions, sliced on the bias

- 2 cups fresh broccoli florets

- 1 cup fresh carrots, shredded

- 2 cups fresh shitake mushrooms, chopped

- 2 tablespoons sesame oil

- 2 teaspoons chili oil

- ½ cup rice wine vinegar

- 2 tablespoons fresh garlic, chopped

- 1 tablespoon fresh ginger, chopped

- ¼ cup low-sodium soy sauce substitute (recipe below)

- ¼ cup fresh lime juice (about 2 limes) and zest of 1 lime (1 tablespoon)

- Low-Sodium Soy Sauce Substitute (makes 1 cup):

- 4 teaspoons Better Than Bouillon®

- Chicken Base (low sodium)

- 1 teaspoon reduced-sodium soy sauce

- 4 teaspoons balsamic vinegar

- 2 teaspoons dark molasses

- ¼ teaspoon ground ginger

- ¼ teaspoon white pepper

- ¼ teaspoon garlic powder

- 1½ cups water

Instructions

1. Combine ingredients for soy sauce substitute in small saucepan.

2. Stir on medium heat. Allow to reduce and thicken slightly to about 1 cup. Store remainder in refrigerator.

3. Then, mix first 6 ingredients together in large bowl and set aside.

4. Blend remaining ingredients together in blender until well incorporated, about 1 minute.

5. Pour dressing mixture over pasta mixture. Toss until well coated, then serve.

Knock-Your-Socks-Off Chicken Broccoli Stromboli

Preparation time

35 minutes

Ingredients

- 1 pound store-bought pizza dough (Note: dough can be purchased at some local pizzerias as well as grocery stores)

- 2 cups fresh broccoli florets, blanched

- 2 cups diced cooked chicken breast

- 1 cup shredded low-salt mozzarella cheese

- 1 tablespoon fresh garlic, chopped

- 1 tablespoon fresh oregano, chopped

- 1 teaspoon crushed red pepper flakes

- 2 tablespoons flour

- 2 tablespoons olive oil

Instructions

1. Preheat oven to 400° F.

2. Mix chicken, cheese, pepper flakes, broccoli, garlic and oregano in large bowl and set aside.

3. Dust tabletop with flour and roll out dough until you reach an 11" x 14" rectangular shape.

4. Place chicken mixture about 2 inches from the edge of the dough, along the longest side.

5. Roll and pinch the ends and seam until tightly sealed (a fork can be used to crimp edges for a tight seal).

6. Brush the top with olive oil and make 3 small slits on the top of the dough.

7. Bake 8–12 minutes or until golden brown on lightly oiled baking sheet tray.

8. Remove, let sit for 3–5 minutes, then slice and serve

Cool and Crispy Cucumber Salad

Preparation time

Ingredients

- 2 cups fresh cucumber (sliced into ¼-inch slices, peeling is optional)

- 2 tablespoons Italian or Caesar salad dressing

- Fresh ground black pepper to taste

Instructions

1. In medium-size bowl with lid, combine cucumber and salad dressing.

2. Cover with lid, shake to coat.

3. Sprinkle with ground black pepper.

4. Refrigerate.

5. Best served cold.

Smoky & Savory Salmon Dip

Preparation time

1 hour 15 minutes

Ingredients

- 1 pound fresh skinless, boneless salmon cut into 4 pieces

- 2 teaspoons smoked paprika

- 1 cup cream cheese

- ¼ cup capers

- ¼ cup lemon juice and zest of half a lemon (about 1 teaspoon)

- 2 tablespoons red onions, finely diced

- 1 teaspoon ground black pepper

- 1 tablespoon fresh parsley, chopped

Instructions

1. Poach the salmon in 2 cups of water and 1 teaspoon of smoked paprika for 4–6 minutes on medium-high heat; the pot should be covered but it should not reach a boil.

2. Remove and chill for at least 30 minutes.

3. Mix all of the other ingredients together until smooth.

4. Break salmon into bite-sized pieces and fold into the cream cheese mixture.

5. Chill salmon dip for 20–30 minutes. Serve with celery sticks, corn chips and carrots or rolled in a leaf of iceberg lettuce.

Herb-Roasted Chicken Breasts

Preparation time

5 hours

Ingredients

• 1 pound boneless, skinless chicken breasts

- 1 medium onion

- 1–2 garlic cloves

- 2 tablespoons Mrs. Dash® Garlic and Herb Seasoning Blend

- 1 teaspoon ground black pepper

- ¼ cup olive oil

Instructions

Marinating:

1. Chop onion and garlic and place in a bowl. Add Mrs. Dash Seasoning, ground pepper and olive oil.

2. Add chicken breasts to the marinade, cover it, then refrigerate for at least 4 hours or overnight.

Baking:

1. Preheat the oven to 350°F.

2. Cover a baking sheet with foil, place the marinated chicken breasts on the pan.

3. Pour the remaining marinade over the chicken and bake at 350°F for 20 minutes.

4. Broil an additional 5 minutes for browning.

Fired-Up Zucchini Turkey Burger

Preparation time

30 minutes

Ingredients

• 1 pound ground turkey meat

• 1 cup zucchini, shredded

• ½ cup onion, minced

• 1 jalapeño pepper, sliced lengthwise, seeded and minced

• 1 egg

• 1 teaspoon Mrs. Dash® Extra Spicy Blend

- 2 fresh poblano peppers, sliced in half lengthwise and seeded

- 1 teaspoon mustard (optional)

Instructions

1. Mix the first 6 ingredients thoroughly.

2. Form meat mixture into 4 turkey burger patties.

3. Turkey burgers may be grilled outdoors on a grill or on an electric griddle.

4. The peppers can be grilled alongside turkey burgers until the skin is tender and blistered.

5. Grill turkey burgers to an internal temperature of 165° F or until center is no longer pink.

6. Top the patty with sliced grilled peppers and serve on a hamburger bun.

Egg Fried Rice

Preparation time

25 minutes

Ingredients

- 2 teaspoons dark sesame oil

- 2 eggs

- 2 egg whites

- 1 tablespoon canola oil

- 1 cup bean sprouts

- ⅓ cup green onions, chopped

- 4 cups cooked rice, cold

- 1 cup frozen peas, thawed

- ¼ teaspoon ground black pepper

Instructions

1. Combine the sesame oil, eggs and egg whites in a small bowl.

2. Stir well and set aside.

3. Heat canola oil in a large nonstick skillet over medium-high heat.

4. Add egg mixture and stir-fry until done.

5. Add bean sprouts and green onions. Stir-fry for 2 minutes.

6. Add rice and peas. Continue to stir-fry until heated thoroughly.

7. Season with black pepper and serve immediately.

Three-Pea Salad with Ginger-Lime Vinaigrette

Preparation time

20 minutes

Ingredients

- 1 cup sugar snap peas

- 1 cup snow peas

- 1 cup fresh or thawed frozen sweet peas

- Vinaigrette:

- 1 teaspoon soy sauce, reduced sodium

- ¼ cup fresh lime juice

- 1 teaspoon fresh lime zest

- 2 teaspoons fresh ginger, chopped

- ½ cup canola oil (can substitute grapeseed oil)

- 1 tablespoon hot sesame oil

- 1 tablespoon sesame seeds

Optional garnish: freshly cracked coarse black pepper to taste

Instructions

1. Lightly toast the sesame seeds in a hot skillet, tossing them constantly for about 3–5 minutes.

2. In a large pot of boiling water over high heat, blanch all 3 types of peas for 2 minutes, drain and then shock them in a bowl of cold water.

3. Transfer to a strainer and drain thoroughly.

4. In a small bowl, whisk the soy sauce, black pepper, lime juice and zest until well-blended, about 1–2 minutes.

5. Continue to whisk, adding the ginger.

6. Slowly drizzle in the canola or grapeseed oil, then add the sesame oil, mixing until well incorporated.

7. In a large bowl, combine the salad dressing with the pea mixture.

8. Toss with the sesame seeds, add the black pepper to taste and serve.

9. Optional: Garnish with freshly cracked coarse black pepper to taste.

Spicy Veggie Vindaloo with Naan

Preparation time

20 minutes

Ingredients

- 2 tablespoons mustard oil, ghee oil or canola oil

- 2 shallots, diced

- ¼ cup eggplant, peeled and diced

- ¼ cup zucchini, diced

- ¼ cup cauliflower

- ½ cup mixed red and green peppers, diced

- 1 cup quinoa, cooked

- 2 tablespoons fresh lime juice

- 2 tablespoons fresh cilantro, chopped

- ½ cup paneer or queso fresco

- 4–6 mini Indian naan bread

- Seasoning mix:

- 2 teaspoons curry powder

- ½ teaspoon turmeric

- ½ teaspoon ground cumin

- ½ teaspoon red chili pepper flakes, ground

- ¼ teaspoon ground cinnamon

- ¼ teaspoon ground cloves

- ¼ teaspoon ground ginger

Optional garnish: 2 tablespoons sour cream and lime wedges

Instructions

1. Cook the quinoa by package directions.

2. Prepare the dry seasoning mix.

3. In a large sauté pan, heat the oil on medium-high, then add the shallots, eggplant, zucchini, cauliflower and mixed peppers and sauté for 2–4 minutes. The vegetables should be slightly translucent and still crunchy. Add the seasoning mix and stir until well-mixed.

4. Turn off heat and stir in the cooked quinoa, lime juice, cilantro and cheese.

5. Serve either hot or cold. TO SERVE HOT: Spread veggie mix evenly on top of warm naan bread. TO SERVE CHILLED: Chill filling. Then add evenly to naan bread.

Optional: May eat with or without Naan bread.

Jalapeño-Lime Turkey Burger with Smoked Mozzarella

Preparation time

20 minutes

Ingredients

- 2 tablespoons jalapeño,* finely diced

- juice of 2 limes and zest** of 1 lime

- 1 tablespoon freshly ground black pepper

- 1 tablespoon French's® Worcestershire sauce, reduced sodium

- 4 tablespoons extra virgin olive oil

- 8 slices of mozzarella cheese with skim milk

- 2 pounds ground turkey

- 8 hamburger buns, toasted

Instructions

1. In a medium-sized bowl, combine the first 5 ingredients plus 2 tablespoons of olive oil.

2. Form 8 equal-sized turkey burger patties and lightly brush them with 2 tablespoons of olive oil.

3. In a large nonstick sauté pan over medium-high heat, heat half of the canola oil on medium-high (a George Foreman® grill may also be used).

4. Cook the burgers for 5–7 minutes per side, flipping once or until an internal temperature of

165° F is reached with an instant-read thermometer.

5. Top each burger with about 2 tablespoons of cheese and melt in a toaster oven or an oven set to broil.

6. Serve each turkey burger on a toasted bun. (If using a George Foreman® grill, once cooked, unplug the grill and add cheese to the burger. Leave the grill open and allow the cheese to slightly melt.)

Pesto-Crusted Catfish

Preparation time

45 minutes

Ingredients

- 2 pounds catfish (boned and filleted) 6 5-ounce pieces

- 4 teaspoons pesto

- ¾ cup panko bread crumbs

- ½ cup mozzarella cheese

- 2 tablespoons olive oil

- 1 teaspoon garlic powder

- 1 teaspoon onion powder

- ½ teaspoon dried oregano

- ½ teaspoon red pepper flakes

- ½ teaspoon black pepper

Instructions

1. Preheat oven to 400° F.

2. Mix all the seasonings in small bowl and begin to sprinkle even amounts on both sides of fish.

3. Spread equal amounts of pesto (1 teaspoon each) on topside of filets and set aside.

4. In medium bowl, mix cheese, oil and bread crumbs and dredge pesto side of fish in mixture until well coated.

5. Grease or spray baking sheet tray liberally with oil and lay fish pesto side up on sheet tray leaving space between filets.

6. Bake for 15–20 minutes at 400° F or until desired brownness on bottom rack.

7. Let rest for 10 minutes after cooking and removing from tray to prevent fish from breaking.

Chili Cornbread Casserole

Preparation time

1 hour 20 minutes

Ingredients

Chili:

- 1 pound ground beef

- ½ cup onions, diced

- ¼ cup celery, diced

- 2 tablespoons jalapeño peppers, chopped

- ½ cup red or green peppers, chopped

- 1 tablespoon chili powder

- 1 tablespoon granulated garlic powder

- 2 tablespoons dried onion flakes

- 1 tablespoon cumin

- 1 teaspoon ground black pepper

- ½ cup tomato sauce, no added salt

- ¼ cup water

- ¼ cup French's® Worcestershire sauce, reduced sodium

- 1 cup kidney beans, rinsed and drained

- 1 cup cheddar cheese, shredded

Cornbread:

- ¼ cup cornmeal

- ¾ cup flour

- ¼ teaspoon baking soda

- ½ teaspoon cream of tartar

- ½ cup sugar

- 1 egg, beaten

- 1½ tablespoons butter, unsalted, melted

- ¼ cup canola oil

- ¾ cup milk

Instructions

1. In a large saucepot, brown ground beef with onions, celery, jalapeños and bell peppers. Drain any excess oil.

2. Add chili powder, garlic powder, onion flakes, cumin, black pepper, tomato sauce, water, Worcestershire sauce and beans.

3. Cook for an additional 10 minutes.

4. Remove from heat and pour into 9" x 9" baking pan, then layer cheese.

5. In a medium-sized bowl, mix cornmeal, flour, baking soda, cream of tartar and sugar.

6. In a small bowl, beat egg, melted butter, oil and milk.

7. Fold flour mixture and egg mixture together (you should see some lumps, which is fine, don't over beat).

8. Pour mixture over chili and bake for 25 minutes uncovered, then 20 minutes covered at 350° F and then turn off oven and let rest for 5 minutes.

Smokin´ Good Chicken With Mustard Sauce

Preparation time

20 minutes

Ingredients

- 2 pounds thinly sliced chicken breast (or boneless skinless chicken breast pounded thin)

- ¼ cup diced shallots

- ¼ cup fresh scallions, chopped

- ½ cup flour

- ½ cup canola oil

- 2 cups low-sodium chicken stock

- 1 tablespoon Better Than Bouillon® Chicken Base (low sodium)

- 2 tablespoons brown mustard

- ½ stick unsalted butter, chilled and cubed

Seasonings:

- ½ teaspoon black pepper

- ½ teaspoon Italian seasoning

- 1 tablespoon dried parsley

- 1 tablespoon smoked paprika

Instructions

1. Mix pepper, Italian seasoning, paprika and parsley in small bowl.

2. Sprinkle half on the chicken breast and add the remainder to flour.

3. Heat oil in large sauté pan on medium-high heat.

4. Remove 3 tablespoons of seasoned flour and set aside.

5. Dredge chicken in remaining seasoned flour and sauté for 2–3 minutes each side.

6. Remove chicken and set aside on a plate to rest. Remove all but a few tablespoons of the oil; add shallots and sauté until slightly translucent.

7. Whisk in flour until smooth and start to gradually add stock while continuing to whisk.

8. After 5 minutes of cooking on medium-high heat, lower heat and whisk in mustard, chicken bouillon and unsalted butter.

9. Turn off heat and return chicken and all juice drippings from plate back to pan and stir.

10. Plate and garnish with scallions

Fall Harvest Orzo Salad

Preparation time

5 minutes

Ingredients

• 4 cups cooked orzo, chilled (about 1 2/3 cups dried orzo)

- 1 cup dried cranberries

- 2 cups fresh apples, diced

- ¼ cup extra-virgin olive oil

- ¼ cup fresh lemon juice

- ½ teaspoon freshly ground black pepper

- 2 tablespoons fresh basil, chopped

- ½ cup crumbled blue cheese

- ¼ cup blanched almonds, chopped

Instructions

1. In a medium-size bowl, add all the ingredients except blue cheese and almonds, gently combining until well incorporated.

2. Transfer the mixture to a serving dish, sprinkle with the crumbled blue cheese and almonds and serve.

Meatloaf

Preparation time

45 minutes

Ingredients

- 1 pound 85% lean ground beef or ground turkey

- 1 egg, beaten

- ½ cup panko bread crumbs

- 2 tablespoons mayonnaise

Seasonings:

- 1 teaspoon garlic powder

- 1 teaspoon onion powder

- 1 teaspoon Better Than Bouillon® Beef Base (low sodium)

- 1 tablespoon low-sodium Worcestershire sauce

- ½ teaspoon red pepper flakes

Instructions

1. Mix all ingredients (except ground beef or turkey) in a medium-size bowl until well incorporated.

2. Add ground beef or turkey and mix.

3. Put mixture into meatloaf pan or form into an 8 "x 4" oblong loaf or desired meatloaf shape or form into 2 individual-size meatloaves and place on a small baking sheet tray.

4. Cover with aluminum foil and bake 20 minutes, then remove foil and cook for an additional 5 minutes.

5. Turn oven off and let rest in oven for 10 minutes before removing and serving.

Crunchy Lemon-Herbed Chicken

Preparation time

20 minutes

Ingredients

- 6 2-ounce chicken tenders

- 4 Tablespoons unsalted butter, chilled

- ½ cup panko bread crumbs

- ¼ cup of lemon juice, plus zest of 1 lemon

- 1 egg yolk

- 1 Tablespoon fresh oregano, chopped

- 1 Tablespoon fresh basil, chopped

- 1 Tablespoon fresh thyme, chopped

- 3 Tablespoons water (1 tablespoon for the egg wash, 2 tablespoons for finishing the sauce)

Instructions

Preheat 2 tablespoons of butter on medium-low heat.

1. Add zest of 1 lemon and half the herbs to bread crumbs, save the rest for lemon sauce.

2. Beat egg yolk with 1 tablespoon water.

3. Place chicken tenders between 2 pieces of plastic wrap and beat with small groove side of mallet until thin, but not ripped.

4. Dip chicken in egg wash mixture, then in herbed bread crumb mixture until coated.

5. Set them aside.

6. Preheat 2 tablespoons of butter on medium heat.

7. Place breaded chicken in sauté pan.

8. Cook chicken, approximately 2–3 minutes each side.

9. Remove chicken and place on baking sheet pan to rest.

10.   In same pan, add remaining herbs and lemon juice, then heat until simmering.

11. Turn off heat; add remaining 2 Tablespoons of butter to the sauce, stir vigorously.

12. Slice the chicken.

13. Place sliced chicken on a plate, pour the sauce over the top and add garnishes.

Bourbon-Glazed Skirt Steak

Preparation time

2 hours

Ingredients

Bourbon Glaze:

• ¼ cup diced shallots

• 3 tablespoons unsalted butter, chilled and cubed

• 1 cup bourbon

• ¼ cup dark brown sugar

• 2 tablespoons Dijon mustard

- 1 tablespoon black pepper

Skirt Steak:

- 2 tablespoons grape seed oil

- ½ teaspoon dried oregano

- ½ teaspoon smoked paprika

- 1 teaspoon black pepper

- 1 tablespoon red wine vinegar

- 2 pounds skirt steak

Instructions

Bourbon Glaze:

1. In small saucepan on medium-high heat, brown shallots in 1 tablespoon butter.

2. Reduce heat to low, remove pan from stove, add bourbon and then place saucepan back on stove.

3. Cook for 10–15 minutes, or until reduced by about one third.

4. Add brown sugar, mustard and black pepper and stir until bubbly.

5. Turn off heat and stir in the remaining 2 tablespoons of cold, cubed butter, stirring constantly until well incorporated.

Skirt Steak:

1. Mix first 5 ingredients in gallon-size sealable storage bag, add steaks and shake well.

2. Allow steaks to marinate in bag at room temperature for 30–45 minutes.

3. Remove steaks from bag, grill for 15– 20 minutes each side, then remove and let rest for 10 minutes.

4. Slice and serve with a drizzle of sauce; or leave whole and brush with glaze and put in preheated broiler for 4–6 minutes, or until desired look.

Pumpkin Strudel

Preparation time

40 minutes

Ingredients

- 1½ cups canned pumpkin, sodium-free, unsweetened

- ⅛ teaspoon grated nutmeg

- 1 teaspoon pure vanilla extract

- 4 tablespoons sugar

- ½ teaspoon ground cinnamon

- ½ stick (4 tablespoons) butter, unsalted, melted

- 12 sheets phyllo dough (follow package directions for defrosting if frozen)

Instructions

1. Position the oven rack in the middle of the oven.

2. Preheat the oven to 375° F.

3. In a medium-sized bowl, combine the canned pumpkin, nutmeg, vanilla extract, 2 tablespoons of sugar and ½ tablespoon of cinnamon until well-mixed.

4. Using a pastry brush, coat the bottom of a nonstick medium sheet tray with the melted butter.

5. On a clean work surface, lay down a single sheet of phyllo dough, and brush it with the butter.

6. Then create a stack of buttered phyllo sheets, brushing every other phyllo sheet with butter. (Be sure to save a little melted butter to brush the top of the rolled filled strudel, so go lightly when brushing in between layers.)

7. Keep remaining phyllo dough sheets covered with plastic wrap until ready for use, so they do not dry out.

8. Once all 12 sheets are used, spoon the mixture evenly along one of the long edges of the stack.

9. Roll from the filled end to the unfilled end, making sure the seam-side faces down.

10. Transfer the roll to the greased sheet tray seam-side down and brush with the remaining butter.

11. In a small bowl, mix the remaining sugar and cinnamon.

12. Sprinkle it over the top and sides of the strudel.

13. Bake on the middle rack until lightly toasted or golden brown, about 12–15 minutes.

14. Remove the tray from the oven and allow the toasted strudel to rest for 5-10 minutes before slicing with a sharp knife, allowing the center to settle.

15. Serve.

Orange and Cinnamon Biscotti

Preparation time

1 hour 30 minutes

Ingredients

- 1 cup sugar

- ½ cup unsalted butter, room temperature

- 2 large eggs

- 2 teaspoons grated orange peel

- 1 teaspoon vanilla extract

- 2 cups all purpose flour

- 1 teaspoon cream of tartar

- ½ teaspoon baking soda

- 1 teaspoon ground cinnamon

- ¼ teaspoon salt

Instructions

1. Preheat oven to 325° F.

2. Spray 2 baking sheets with nonstick cooking spray.

3. Beat sugar and unsalted butter in a large bowl until well blended.

4. Add eggs one at a time, beating well after each.

5. Beat in orange peel and vanilla.

6. Mix flour, cream of tartar, baking soda, cinnamon and salt in a medium-size bowl.

7. Add dry ingredients to butter mixture and mix until incorporated.

8. Divide dough in half.

9. Place each half on a prepared sheet.

10. With lightly floured hands, form each half into a log shape that is 3 inches wide by three quarters of an inch high.

11. Bake until dough logs are firm to the touch, about 35 minutes.

12. Remove dough logs from oven and cool 10 minutes.

13. Transfer logs to work surface. Using serrated knife, cut on diagonal into ½-inch-thick slices.

14. Arrange cut side down on baking sheets.

15. Bake until bottoms are golden, about 12 minutes.

16. Turn biscotti over; bake until bottoms are golden, about 12 minutes longer.

17. Transfer to a wire rack and cool before serving.

Dry-Rubbed Barbecue Turkey Wings

Preparation time

1 hour 20 minutes

Ingredients

- 7 whole turkey wings

- Chef McCargo's Barbecue Spice Rub (mix all ingredients together):

- 1 cup packed dark brown sugar

- 1 teaspoon black pepper

- 1 teaspoon red pepper flakes

- 1 teaspoon smoked paprika

- 2 teaspoons granulated garlic

- 2 teaspoons dehydrated onion flakes

- 2 teaspoons dark chili powder

- 14 tablespoons of your favorite low-sodium barbecue sauce (2 tablespoons per wing)

Instructions

1. Preheat oven to 375° F.

2. Pat wings dry and pierce with fork on both sides.

3. Rub wings liberally with spice rub, saving 1 tablespoon for later.

4. Place wings on baking sheet tray and bake wrapped with foil for 30 minutes.

5. Remove wings from oven and discard foil, flip over and cook for an additional 30 minutes.

6. Sprinkle rest of seasoning on wings and flip back over.

7. Turn off oven and let wings sit in oven for 15 minutes, then serve with a side of low-sodium barbecue sauce.

Sweet Cornbread Muffins With Citrus Honey Butter

Preparation time

35 minutes

Ingredients

- 1 cup cornmeal

- 1 cup flour

- 1 ½ teaspoons baking soda

- 3 tablespoons lemon juice

- 1 egg, beaten

- 1 cup milk

- ½ stick unsalted butter, melted

- 1 tablespoon vanilla extract

Honey Butter:

- 2 tablespoons honey

- 1 stick unsalted butter, softened

- ½ teaspoon orange zest

- ¼ teaspoon black pepper

- ½ teaspoon orange extract

Instructions

1. Preheat oven to 400° F.

2. In a large bowl, beat egg, milk and butter together until mixed well.

3. In a separate bowl, mix flour, cornmeal and baking soda, then fold into liquid ingredients until smooth. Be sure not to overbeat.

4. Line muffin tins with muffin liner, fill each cup ¾ full and bake for 15–20 minutes on middle rack.

5. In a small bowl, whisk honey butter ingredients until blended; spread on top of

cornbread muffins or serve honey butter on the side.

Chocolate Smoothie

Preparation time

5 minutes

Ingredients

* 2 scoops chocolate-flavored whey protein

* 2 cups ice

* 2 tablespoons Southern Comfort® liqueur (optional)

* ½ cup evaporated milk

- ¼ cup condensed milk

- ¼ teaspoon ground cinnamon

- Pinch of nutmeg

Instructions

1. Mix all ingredients except cinnamon in blender on high until smooth, approximately 1–2 minutes.

2. Top with whipped cream and sprinkle with cinnamon to garnish.

Heavenly Deviled Eggs

Preparation time

10 minutes

Ingredients

- 4 large eggs, hard boiled with shells removed

- 2 tablespoons light mayonnaise

- ½ teaspoon dry mustard

- ½ teaspoon cider vinegar

- 1 tablespoon onion, finely chopped

- ¼ teaspoon ground black pepper

Optional garnish: dash of paprika

Instructions

1. Cut eggs in half, lengthwise.

2. Carefully remove yolks and place in a small bowl.

3. Place egg white on a plate.

4. Mash yolks with a fork and mix in dry mustard, vinegar, onion and ground black pepper.

5. Reflll cooked egg white with yolk mixture, heaping slightly.

6. Sprinkle deviled eggs with paprika (optional) and serve.

9 798715 662644